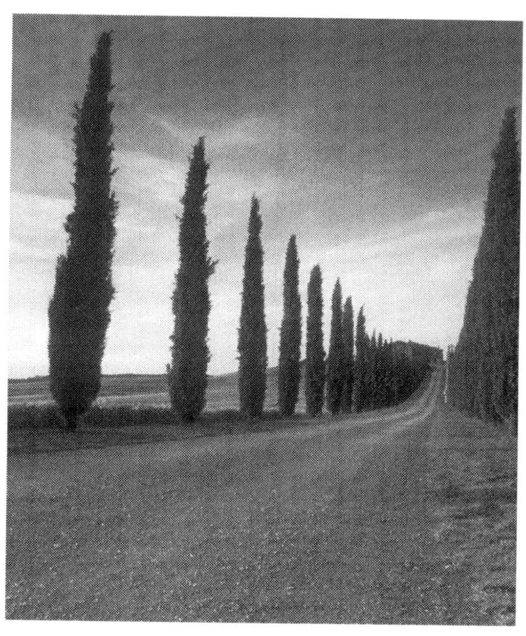

SYMPTOM JOURNAL

Fatigue and Symptom Tracker

CFS
ME
MS
FIBROMYALGI
A LUPUS
SYMPTOM
JOURNAL

Daily Diary

Use this diary in the way that is most useful to you. It is a simple but comprehensive way of keeping a useful record. Some or all of the sections will be relevant at different points as these chronic conditions fluctuate as do the symptoms experienced. One week you may only experience one or two of the available symptom sections, other weeks you may find most of the sections applicable.

However you use your Journal, I hope you find it is a very useful tool.

AN IDEAL DIARY TO NOTE DOWN SYMPTOMS.

IT CAN BE VERY FRUSTRATING TO ARRIVE FOR YOUR G.P / CONSULTANT APPOINTMENT AND THEN FORGETTING TO MENTION RELEVANT INFORMATION ABOUT YOUR SYMPTOMS.

THIS SIMPLE JOURNAL HAS VARIOUS SECTIONS PER DAY TO ALLOW YOU TO CHRONICLE SYMPTOMS AS AND WHEN THEY OCCUR. HOPEFULLY THIS WILL HELP YOU AND YOUR MEDICAL TEAM MANAGE YOUR HEALTH BY KEEPING ACCURATE RECORDS.

TAKE IT ALONG TO YOUR APPOINTMENT TO REFER TO IF YOU FEEL YOUR MEMORY NEEDS PROMPTING.

HANDY SECTIONS THAT RELATE TO VARIOUS ISSUES PEOPLE WITH CFS / ME/ MS AND LUPUS MAY EXPERIENCE.

MARK PROBLEM AREAS ON BODY DIAGRAM.

Contents:

Use the following to highlight any Journal entry dates for easy future reference:

Date:	Reference: e.g. bad day	page:
Date:	Reference:	page:
Date:	Reference:	page:
Date:	Reference:	page:
Date:	Reference:	page:
Date:	Reference:	page:
Date:	Reference:	page:
Date:	Reference:	page:
Date:	Reference:	page:
Date:	Reference:	page:

Appointment Diary

Doctor's Appointment. Date/Time:	Name of Consultant/Doctor Nurse/Physio	Type: G.P; Neurologist; Rheumatologist Physio Etc.	Reason for appointment: Blood Tests MRI Etc.

Test Results Table

Test Results Date/Time:	Blood Test Name: i.e.: Vit D, ANA, FBC Etc.	Other Test Results. MRI, Scan, EMG, Cardio ETC. *Notes section below table for more space*

Notes regarding test results:

Test Results Table

Test Results Date/Time:	Blood Test Name: i.e.: Vit D, ANA, FBC Etc.	Other Test Results. MRI, Scan, EMG, Cardio ETC. *Notes section below table for more space*

Notes regarding test results:

Prescriptions and treatments

Prescription Date:	Name of medication:	Reason for prescription: pain/infection Etc.	Side Effects if any.	Does it help? Scale 0-10

Notes regarding treatments, therapies or medication:____

Prescriptions and treatments

Prescription Date:	Name of medication:	Reason for prescription: pain/infection Etc.	Side Effects if any.	Does it help? Scale 0-10

Notes regarding treatments, therapies or medication:___________________________________

Fatigue and Symptom Tracker

Day_______________ Date_________

Scale of fatigue 0 = fine, 10 = extremely tired*: note level of fatigue below during your day*

0---------1---------2----------3---------4--------5----------6---------7--------8--------9---------10

Morning:_______ Afternoon:_______ Evening:_______

<u>Cognitive issues</u>: e.g. memory, speech (word forming), comprehension (processing what people are saying) etc.

Write down how it presented itself:

____

____

____

____

____

____

<u>Muscle weakness</u>: jaw, neck, arms (upper/lower), shoulders, lower back/abdomen, hips, legs, swallowing difficulties, head drop:

Activity at time:

____

____

____

____

____

____

<u>Chest and/ or central back pain</u>: activity at time if any; how long it lasted; where exactly and how it presented itself:____

____

____

____

____

____

Daily Diary

Shortness of breath: write activity or when lying down; type of breathlessness:

____

____

____

____

____

____

____

Numbness and tingling/crawling ant sensation: hands; both, one, half, lasted? Feet, toes, lower leg,
other:____

____

____

____

____

____

Balance: try to mark down how often you tipped/wobbled/fell and activity at the
time:____

____

____

____

Bathed: Shower, bath or sink wash.

Yes	No

Result: i.e., breathlessness, pain, muscle fatigue, after
effects:____

Activity: cooking, talking, housework, washing dishes, going out, how many breaks to wash dishes, cook meal, after effects:

____

____

____

____

____

____

____

Notes: other pain or symptoms/medication/eye symptoms, etc:______________________________________

____

____

____

Use the diagram below to indicate area of pain and/or weakness.

Diagram: B: Muscle burning

N: Numbness

CP: Chest and central back pain

MW: Muscle weakness

S: Stiffness (draw an arrow and write letter for symptom)

Above letters are examples, use your own Abbreviations for symptoms not mentioned above.

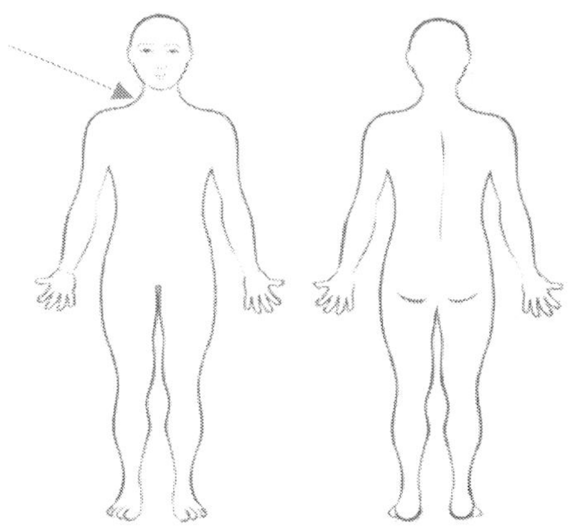

Daily Diary

Day_______________ Date_________

Scale of fatigue 0= fine, 10= extremely tired*: note level of fatigue below during your day*

0---------1---------2----------3---------4--------5----------6---------7--------8--------9---------10

Morning:_______ Afternoon:_______ Evening:_______

Cognitive issues: memory, speech (word forming), comprehension (processing what people are saying)

Write down how it presented itself:

____

____

____

____

____

____

Muscle weakness: jaw, neck, arms (upper/lower), shoulders, lower back/abdomen, hips, legs, swallowing difficulties, head drop:

Activity at time:

____

____

____

____

____

____

Chest and/ or central back pain: activity at time if any; how long it lasted; where exactly and how it presented itself:____

____

____

____

____

____

Shortness of breath: write activity or when lying down; when pulse raised, type of breathlessness:

____
____
____
____
____
____
____

Numbness and tingling/crawling ant sensation: hands; both, one, half, lasted? Feet, toes, lower leg, other:____
____
____
____
____
____

Balance: try to mark down how often you tipped/wobbled/fell and activity at time:____
____
____
____
____
____

Bathed: Shower, bath or sink wash.

Yes	No

Result: i.e., breathlessness, pain, muscle fatigue, after effects:____

Daily Diary

Activity: cooking; talking; housework; washing dishes, going out, how many breaks to wash dishes, cook meal, after effects:

____

____

____

____

____

____

Notes:____

____

____

____

Use the diagram below to indicate area of pain and/or weakness.

Diagram: B: Muscle burning

N: Numbness

CP: Chest and central back pain

MW: Muscle weakness

S: Stiffness (draw an arrow and write letter for symptom)

Above letters are examples, use your own Abbreviations for symptoms not mentioned above.

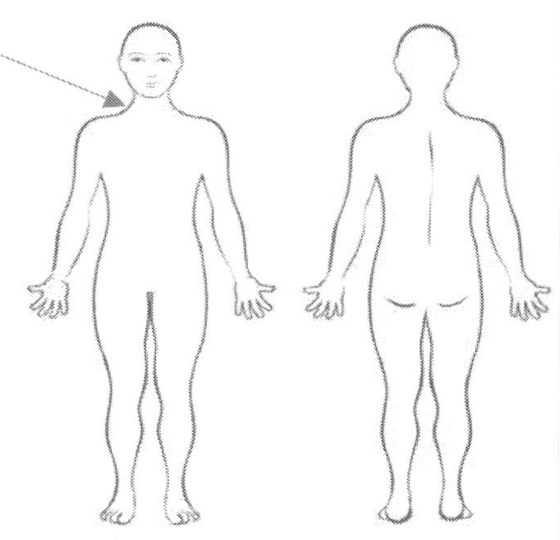

Fatigue and Symptom Tracker

Day________________ Date__________

Scale of fatigue 0= fine, 10= extremely tired*: note level of fatigue below during your day*

0---------1---------2----------3---------4--------5----------6---------7--------8--------9---------10

Morning:_______ Afternoon:_______ Evening:_______

Cognitive issues: memory, speech (word forming), comprehension (processing what people are saying)

Write down how it presented itself:

____

____

____

____

____

____

Muscle weakness: jaw, neck, arms (upper/lower), shoulders, lower back/abdomen, hips, legs, swallowing difficulties, head drop:

Activity at time:

____

____

____

____

____

____

Chest and/ or central back pain: activity at time if any; how long it lasted; where exactly and how it presented itself:____

____

____

____

____

____

Daily Diary

Shortness of breath: write activity or when lying down; when pulse raised, type of breathlessness:

Numbness and tingling/crawling ant sensation: hands; both, one, half, lasted? Feet, toes, lower leg, other:

Balance: try to mark down how often you tipped/wobbled/fell and activity at time:

Bathed: Shower, bath or sink wash.

Yes	No

Result: i.e., breathlessness, pain, muscle fatigue, after effects:

Fatigue and Symptom Tracker

Activity: cooking; talking; housework; washing dishes, going out, how many breaks to wash dishes, cook meal, after effects:

____

____

____

____

____

____

____

Notes:____

____

____

____

Use the diagram below to indicate area of pain and/or weakness.

Diagram: B: Muscle burning

N: Numbness

CP: Chest and central back pain

MW: Muscle weakness

S: Stiffness (draw an arrow and write letter for symptom)

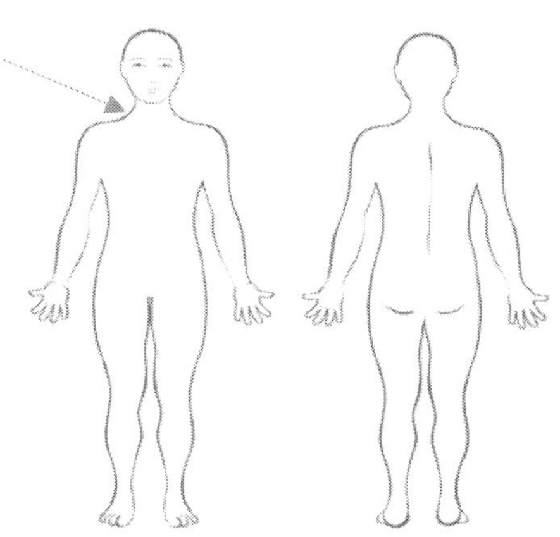

Daily Diary

Day_______________ Date_________

Scale of fatigue 0= fine, 10= extremely tired*: note level of fatigue below during your day*

0---------1---------2---------3---------4--------5----------6---------7--------8--------9---------10

Morning:_______ Afternoon:_______ Evening:_______

<u>Cognitive issues</u>: memory, speech (word forming), comprehension (processing what people are saying)

Write down how it presented itself:

____

____

____

____

____

____

<u>Muscle weakness</u>: jaw, neck, arms (upper/lower), shoulders, lower back/abdomen, hips, legs, swallowing difficulties, head drop:

Activity at time:

____

____

____

____

____

____

<u>Chest and/ or central back pain</u>: activity at time if any; how long it lasted; where exactly and how it presented itself:____

____

____

____

____

____

<u>Shortness of breath</u>: write activity or when lying down; when pulse raised, type of breathlessness:

____
____
____
____
____
____
____

<u>Numbness and tingling/crawling ant sensation</u>: hands; both, one, half, lasted? Feet, toes, lower leg,
other:____
____
____
____
____
____

<u>Balance:</u> try to mark down how often you tipped/wobbled/fell and activity at
time:____
____
____
____
____
____

<u>Bathed: Shower, bath or sink wash.</u>

Yes	No

Result: i.e., breathlessness, pain, muscle fatigue, after
effects:______________________________________

Daily Diary

Activity: cooking; talking; housework; washing dishes, going out, how many breaks to wash dishes, cook meal, after effects:

____

Notes:____

Use the diagram below to indicate area of pain and/or weakness.

Diagram: B: Muscle burning

N: Numbness

CP: Chest and central back pain

MW: Muscle weakness

S: Stiffness (draw an arrow and write letter for symptom)

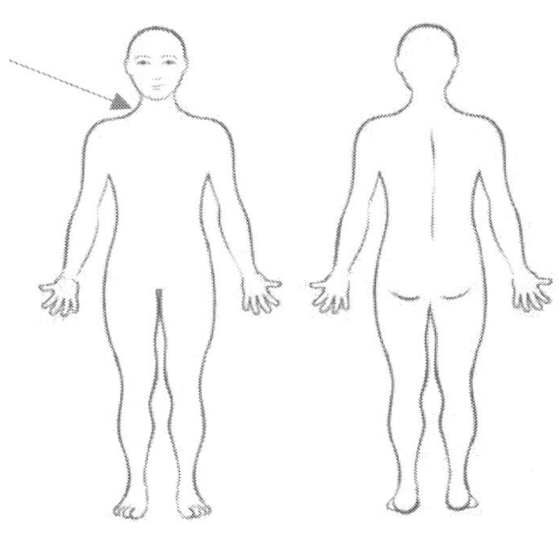

Fatigue and Symptom Tracker

Day_______________ Date_________

Scale of fatigue 0= fine, 10= extremely tired*: note level of fatigue below during your day*

0---------1---------2----------3---------4--------5----------6---------7--------8--------9---------10

Morning:_______ Afternoon:_______ Evening:_______

<u>Cognitive issues</u>: memory, speech (word forming), comprehension (processing what people are saying)

Write down how it presented itself:

____

____

____

____

____

____

<u>Muscle weakness</u>: jaw, neck, arms (upper/lower), shoulders, lower back/abdomen, hips, legs, swallowing difficulties, head drop:

Activity at time:

____

____

____

____

____

____

<u>Chest and/ or central back pain</u>: activity at time if any; how long it lasted; where exactly and how it presented itself:____

____

____

____

____

____

Shortness of breath: write activity or when lying down; when pulse raised, type of breathlessness:

Numbness and tingling/crawling ant sensation: hands; both, one, half, lasted? Feet, toes, lower leg, other:

Balance: try to mark down how often you tipped/wobbled/fell and activity at time:

Bathed: Shower, bath or sink wash.

Yes	No

Result: i.e., breathlessness, pain, muscle fatigue, after effects:

Fatigue and Symptom Tracker

Activity: cooking; talking; housework; washing dishes, going out, how many breaks to wash dishes, cook meal, after effects:

Notes:

Use the diagram below to indicate area of pain and/or weakness.

Diagram: B: Muscle burning

N: Numbness

CP: Chest and central back pain

MW: Muscle weakness

S: Stiffness (draw an arrow and write letter for symptom)

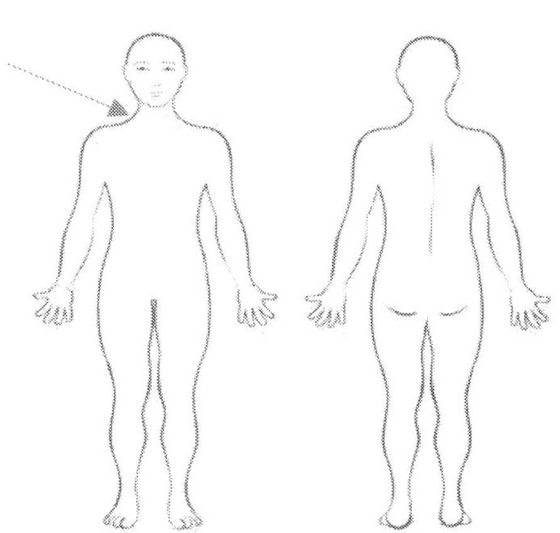

Daily Diary

Day_______________ Date_________

Scale of fatigue 0= fine, 10= extremely tired*: note level of fatigue below during your day*

0---------1---------2----------3---------4--------5----------6---------7--------8--------9---------10

Morning:_______ Afternoon:_______ Evening:_______

Cognitive issues: memory, speech (word forming), comprehension (processing what people are saying)

Write down how it presented itself:

____

____

____

____

____

____

Muscle weakness: jaw, neck, arms (upper/lower), shoulders, lower back/abdomen, hips, legs, swallowing difficulties, head drop:

Activity at time:

____

____

____

____

____

____

Chest and/ or central back pain: activity at time if any; how long it lasted; where exactly and how it presented itself:____

____

____

____

____

____

Shortness of breath: write activity or when lying down; when pulse raised, type of breathlessness:

____

Numbness and tingling/crawling ant sensation: hands; both, one, half, lasted? Feet, toes, lower leg, other:__________________________________

Balance: try to mark down how often you tipped/wobbled/fell and activity at time:__________________________________

Bathed: Shower, bath or sink wash.

Yes	No

Result: i.e., breathlessness, pain, muscle fatigue, after effects:__________________________________

Daily Diary

<u>Activity</u>: cooking; talking; housework; washing dishes, going out, how many breaks to wash dishes, cook meal, after effects:

____

____

____

____

____

____

____

Notes:____

____

____

____

Use the diagram below to indicate area of pain and/or weakness.

Diagram: B: Muscle burning

N: Numbness

CP: Chest and central back pain

MW: Muscle weakness

S: Stiffness (draw an arrow and write letter for symptom)

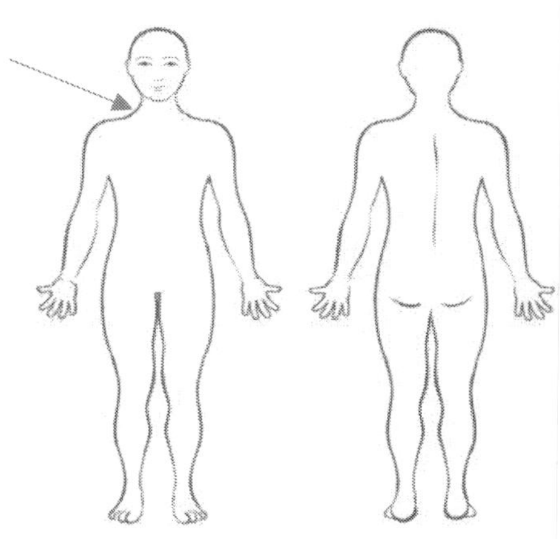

Fatigue and Symptom Tracker

Day________________ Date_________

Scale of fatigue 0= fine, 10= extremely tired*: note level of fatigue below during your day*

0---------1---------2----------3---------4--------5----------6---------7--------8--------9---------10

Morning:_______ Afternoon:_______ Evening:_______

<u>Cognitive issues</u>: memory, speech (word forming), comprehension (processing what people are saying)

Write down how it presented itself:

____
____
____
____
____
____

<u>Muscle weakness</u>: jaw, neck, arms (upper/lower), shoulders, lower back/abdomen, hips, legs, swallowing difficulties, head drop:

Activity at time:

____
____
____
____
____
____

<u>Chest and/ or central back pain</u>: activity at time if any; how long it lasted; where exactly and how it presented itself:____

____
____
____
____
____

Daily Diary

<u>Shortness of breath</u>: write activity or when lying down; when pulse raised, type of breathlessness:

____

____

____

____

____

____

____

<u>Numbness and tingling/crawling ant sensation</u>: hands; both, one, half, lasted? Feet, toes, lower leg, other:_______________________________________

____

____

____

____

____

<u>Balance:</u> try to mark down how often you tipped/wobbled/fell and activity at time:____

____

____

____

____

____

<u>Bathed: Shower, bath or sink wash.</u>

Yes	No

Result: i.e., breathlessness, pain, muscle fatigue, after effects:_______________________________________

Fatigue and Symptom Tracker

Activity: cooking; talking; housework; washing dishes, going out, how many breaks to wash dishes, cook meal, after effects:

____

____

____

____

____

____

____

Notes:____

____

____

____

Use the diagram below to indicate area of pain and/or weakness.

Diagram: B: Muscle burning

N: Numbness

CP: Chest and central back pain

MW: Muscle weakness

S: Stiffness (draw an arrow and write letter for symptom)

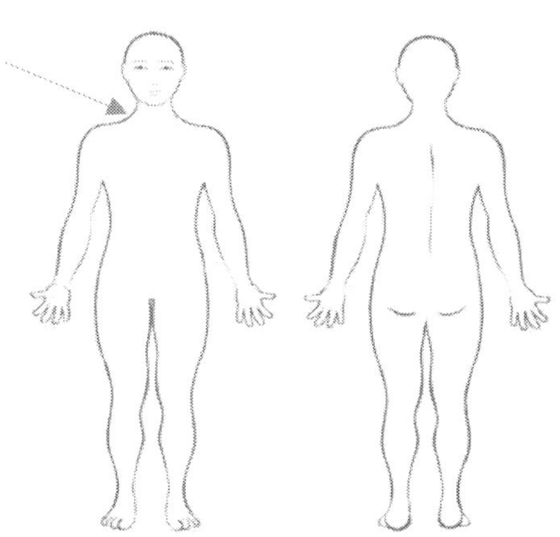

Daily Diary

Day________________ Date__________

Scale of fatigue 0= fine, 10= extremely tired*: note level of fatigue below during your day*

0---------1---------2----------3---------4--------5----------6---------7--------8--------9---------10

Morning:________ Afternoon:________ Evening:________

Cognitive issues: memory, speech (word forming), comprehension (processing what people are saying)

Write down how it presented itself:

____

____

____

____

____

____

Muscle weakness: jaw, neck, arms (upper/lower), shoulders, lower back/abdomen, hips, legs, swallowing difficulties, head drop:

Activity at time:

____

____

____

____

____

____

Chest and/ or central back pain: activity at time if any; how long it lasted; where exactly and how it presented itself:____

____

____

____

____

____

<u>Shortness of breath</u>: write activity or when lying down; when pulse raised, type of breathlessness:

____
____
____
____
____
____
____

<u>Numbness and tingling/crawling ant sensation</u>: hands; both, one, half, lasted? Feet, toes, lower leg, other:____
____
____
____
____
____

<u>Balance:</u> try to mark down how often you tipped/wobbled/fell and activity at time:____
____
____
____
____
____

<u>Bathed: Shower, bath or sink wash.</u>

Yes	No

Result: i.e., breathlessness, pain, muscle fatigue, after effects:____

Daily Diary

Activity: cooking; talking; housework; washing dishes, going out, how many breaks to wash dishes, cook meal, after effects:

____

____

____

____

____

____

____

Notes:____

____

____

____

Use the diagram below to indicate area of pain and/or weakness.

Diagram: B: Muscle burning

N: Numbness

CP: Chest and central back pain

MW: Muscle weakness

S: Stiffness (draw an arrow and write letter for symptom)

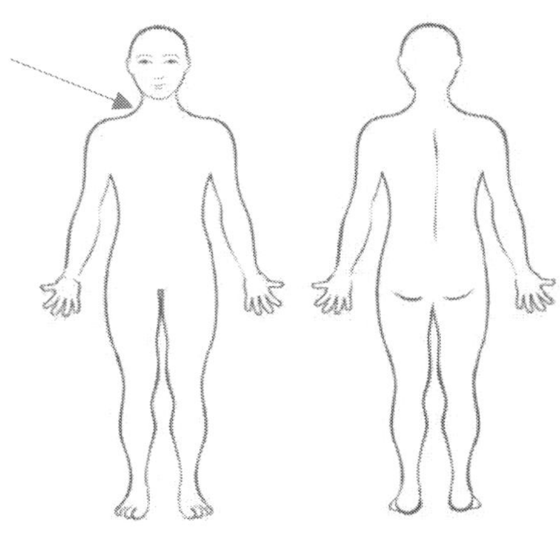

Fatigue and Symptom Tracker

Day________________ Date_________

Scale of fatigue 0= fine, 10= extremely tired: *note level of fatigue below during your day*

0---------1---------2----------3---------4--------5----------6---------7--------8--------9---------10

Morning:_______ Afternoon:_______ Evening:_______

Cognitive issues: memory, speech (word forming), comprehension (processing what people are saying)

Write down how it presented itself:

____

____

____

____

____

____

Muscle weakness: jaw, neck, arms (upper/lower), shoulders, lower back/abdomen, hips, legs, swallowing difficulties, head drop:

Activity at time:

____

____

____

____

____

____

Chest and/ or central back pain: activity at time if any; how long it lasted; where exactly and how it presented itself:____

____

____

____

____

____

Daily Diary

<u>Shortness of breath</u>: write activity or when lying down; when pulse raised, type of breathlessness:

____

Numbness and tingling/crawling ant sensation: hands; both, one, half, lasted? Feet, toes, lower leg, other:

Balance: try to mark down how often you tipped/wobbled/fell and activity at time:

Bathed: Shower, bath or sink wash.

Yes	No

Result: i.e., breathlessness, pain, muscle fatigue, after effects:

Fatigue and Symptom Tracker

Activity: cooking; talking; housework; washing dishes, going out, how many breaks to wash dishes, cook meal, after effects:

Notes:

Use the diagram below to indicate area of pain and/or weakness.

Diagram: B: Muscle burning

N: Numbness

CP: Chest and central back pain

MW: Muscle weakness

S: Stiffness (draw an arrow and write letter for symptom)

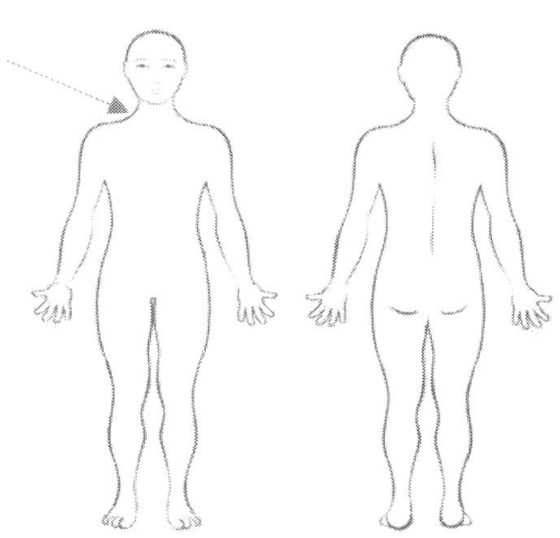

Daily Diary

Day_______________ Date_________

Scale of fatigue 0= fine, 10= extremely tired*: note level of fatigue below during your day*

0---------1---------2----------3---------4--------5----------6---------7--------8--------9---------10

Morning:_______ Afternoon:_______ Evening:_______

Cognitive issues: memory, speech (word forming), comprehension (processing what people are saying)

Write down how it presented itself:

____

____

____

____

____

____

Muscle weakness: jaw, neck, arms (upper/lower), shoulders, lower back/abdomen, hips, legs, swallowing difficulties, head drop:

Activity at time:

____

____

____

____

____

____

Chest and/ or central back pain: activity at time if any; how long it lasted; where exactly and how it presented itself:____

____

____

____

____

____

Shortness of breath: write activity or when lying down; when pulse raised, type of breathlessness:

____
____
____
____
____
____
____

Numbness and tingling/crawling ant sensation: hands; both, one, half, lasted? Feet, toes, lower leg, other:______________________________________

____
____
____
____
____

Balance: try to mark down how often you tipped/wobbled/fell and activity at time:______________________________________

____
____
____
____
____

Bathed: Shower, bath or sink wash.

Yes	No

Result: i.e., breathlessness, pain, muscle fatigue, after effects:______________________________________

Daily Diary

<u>Activity</u>: cooking; talking; housework; washing dishes, going out, how many breaks to wash dishes, cook meal, after effects:

____

____

____

____

____

____

____

Notes:____

____

____

____

Use the diagram below to indicate area of pain and/or weakness.

Diagram: B: Muscle burning

N: Numbness

CP: Chest and central back pain

MW: Muscle weakness

S: Stiffness (draw an arrow and write letter for symptom)

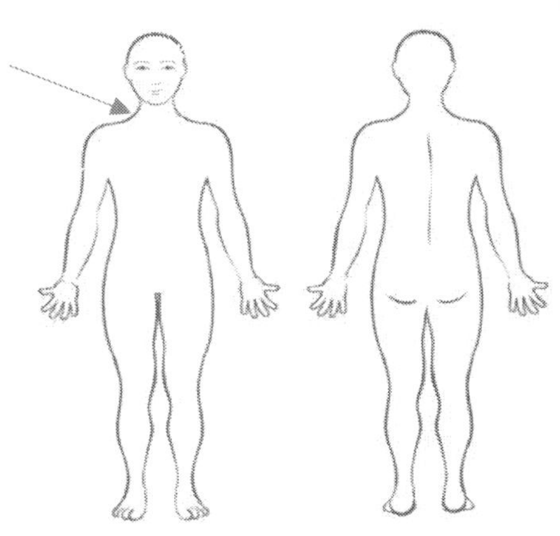

Fatigue and Symptom Tracker

Day________________ Date__________

Scale of fatigue 0= fine, 10= extremely tired*: note level of fatigue below during your day*

0---------1---------2----------3---------4--------5----------6---------7--------8--------9---------10

Morning:________ Afternoon:________ Evening:________

Cognitive issues: memory, speech (word forming), comprehension (processing what people are saying)

Write down how it presented itself:

____

____

____

____

____

____

Muscle weakness: jaw, neck, arms (upper/lower), shoulders, lower back/abdomen, hips, legs, swallowing difficulties, head drop:

Activity at time:

____

____

____

____

____

____

Chest and/ or central back pain: activity at time if any; how long it lasted; where exactly and how it presented itself:____

____

____

____

____

____

Daily Diary

Shortness of breath: write activity or when lying down; when pulse raised, type of breathlessness:

Numbness and tingling/crawling ant sensation: hands; both, one, half, lasted? Feet, toes, lower leg, other:

Balance: try to mark down how often you tipped/wobbled/fell and activity at time:

Bathed: Shower, bath or sink wash.

Yes	No

Result: i.e., breathlessness, pain, muscle fatigue, after effects:

Fatigue and Symptom Tracker

Activity: cooking; talking; housework; washing dishes, going out, how many breaks to wash dishes, cook meal, after effects:

____

____

____

____

____

____

____

Notes:____

____

____

____

Use the diagram below to indicate area of pain and/or weakness.

Diagram: B: Muscle burning

N: Numbness

CP: Chest and central back pain

MW: Muscle weakness

S: Stiffness (draw an arrow and write letter for symptom)

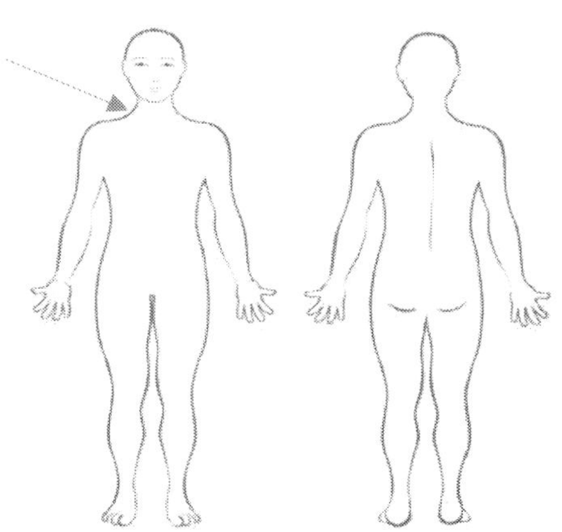

Daily Diary

Day_______________ Date_________

Scale of fatigue 0= fine, 10= extremely tired*: note level of fatigue below during your day*

0---------1---------2----------3---------4--------5----------6---------7--------8--------9---------10

Morning:_______ Afternoon:_______ Evening:_______

Cognitive issues: memory, speech (word forming), comprehension (processing what people are saying)

Write down how it presented itself:

____

____

____

____

____

____

Muscle weakness: jaw, neck, arms (upper/lower), shoulders, lower back/abdomen, hips, legs, swallowing difficulties, head drop:

Activity at time:

____

____

____

____

____

____

Chest and/ or central back pain: activity at time if any; how long it lasted; where exactly and how it presented itself:____

____

____

____

____

____

Shortness of breath: write activity or when lying down; when pulse raised, type of breathlessness:

____

____

____

____

____

____

____

Numbness and tingling/crawling ant sensation: hands; both, one, half, lasted? Feet, toes, lower leg, other:____

____

____

____

____

____

Balance: try to mark down how often you tipped/wobbled/fell and activity at time:____

____

____

____

____

____

Bathed: Shower, bath or sink wash.

Yes	No

Result: i.e., breathlessness, pain, muscle fatigue, after effects:____

____

Daily Diary

<u>Activity</u>: cooking; talking; housework; washing dishes, going out, how many breaks to wash dishes, cook meal, after effects:

____

____

____

____

____

____

____

Notes:____

____

____

____

Use the diagram below to indicate area of pain and/or weakness.

Diagram: B: Muscle burning

N: Numbness

CP: Chest and central back pain

MW: Muscle weakness

S: Stiffness (draw an arrow and write letter for symptom)

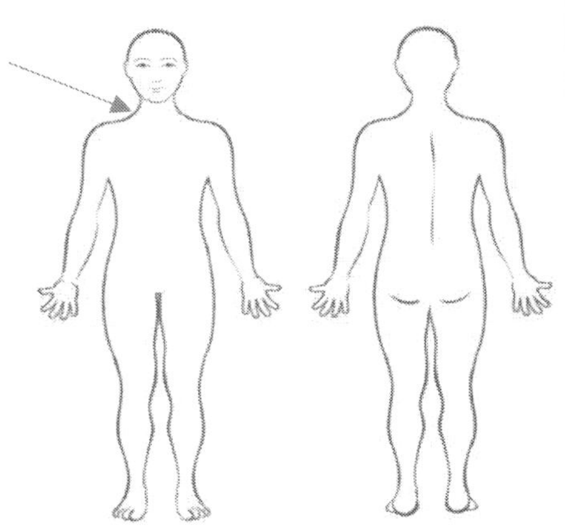

Fatigue and Symptom Tracker

Day________________ Date__________

Scale of fatigue 0= fine, 10= extremely tired*: note level of fatigue below during your day*

0---------1---------2----------3---------4--------5----------6---------7--------8--------9---------10

Morning:________ Afternoon:________ Evening:________

<u>Cognitive issues</u>: memory, speech (word forming), comprehension (processing what people are saying)

Write down how it presented itself:

____

____

____

____

____

____

<u>Muscle weakness</u>: jaw, neck, arms (upper/lower), shoulders, lower back/abdomen, hips, legs, swallowing difficulties, head drop:

Activity at time:

____

____

____

____

____

____

<u>Chest and/ or central back pain</u>: activity at time if any; how long it lasted; where exactly and how it presented itself:____

____

____

____

____

____

Shortness of breath: write activity or when lying down; when pulse raised, type of breathlessness:

____

Numbness and tingling/crawling ant sensation: hands; both, one, half, lasted? Feet, toes, lower leg, other:____

Balance: try to mark down how often you tipped/wobbled/fell and activity at time:____

Bathed: Shower, bath or sink wash.

Yes	No

Result: i.e., breathlessness, pain, muscle fatigue, after effects:____

Fatigue and Symptom Tracker

Activity: cooking; talking; housework; washing dishes, going out, how many breaks to wash dishes, cook meal, after effects:

____

Notes:____

Use the diagram below to indicate area of pain and/or weakness.

Diagram: B: Muscle burning

N: Numbness

CP: Chest and central back pain

MW: Muscle weakness

S: Stiffness (draw an arrow and write letter for symptom)

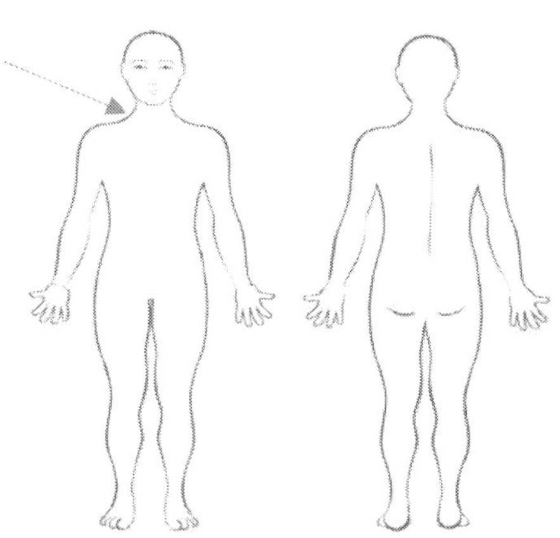

Daily Diary

Day_______________ Date_________

Scale of fatigue 0= fine, 10= extremely tired*: note level of fatigue below during your day*

0---------1---------2----------3---------4--------5----------6---------7--------8--------9---------10

Morning:_______ Afternoon:_______ Evening:_______

Cognitive issues: memory, speech (word forming), comprehension (processing what people are saying)

Write down how it presented itself:

____

____

____

____

____

____

Muscle weakness: jaw, neck, arms (upper/lower), shoulders, lower back/abdomen, hips, legs, swallowing difficulties, head drop:

Activity at time:

____

____

____

____

____

____

Chest and/ or central back pain: activity at time if any; how long it lasted; where exactly and how it presented itself:____

____

____

____

____

____

Shortness of breath: write activity or when lying down; when pulse raised, type of breathlessness:

Numbness and tingling/crawling ant sensation: hands; both, one, half, lasted? Feet, toes, lower leg, other:

Balance: try to mark down how often you tipped/wobbled/fell and activity at time:

Bathed: Shower, bath or sink wash.

Yes	No

Result: i.e., breathlessness, pain, muscle fatigue, after effects:

Daily Diary

Activity: cooking; talking; housework; washing dishes, going out, how many breaks to wash dishes, cook meal, after effects:

____

____

____

____

____

____

____

Notes:____

____

____

____

Use the diagram below to indicate area of pain and/or weakness.

Diagram: B: Muscle burning

N: Numbness

CP: Chest and central back pain

MW: Muscle weakness

S: Stiffness (draw an arrow and write letter for symptom)

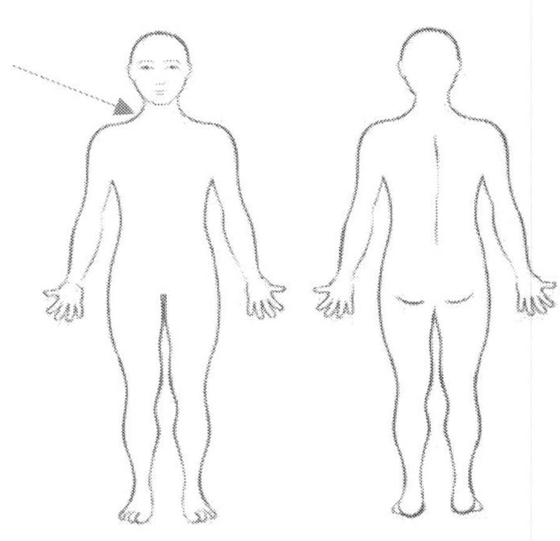

Fatigue and Symptom Tracker

Day________________ Date__________

Scale of fatigue 0= fine, 10= extremely tired*: note level of fatigue below during your day*

0---------1---------2----------3---------4--------5----------6---------7--------8--------9---------10

Morning:________ Afternoon:________ Evening:________

Cognitive issues: memory, speech (word forming), comprehension (processing what people are saying)

Write down how it presented itself:

____

____

____

____

____

____

Muscle weakness: jaw, neck, arms (upper/lower), shoulders, lower back/abdomen, hips, legs, swallowing difficulties, head drop:

Activity at time:

____

____

____

____

____

____

Chest and/ or central back pain: activity at time if any; how long it lasted; where exactly and how it presented itself:____

____

____

____

____

____

Shortness of breath: write activity or when lying down; when pulse raised, type of breathlessness:

Numbness and tingling/crawling ant sensation: hands; both, one, half, lasted? Feet, toes, lower leg, other:

Balance: try to mark down how often you tipped/wobbled/fell and activity at time:

Bathed: Shower, bath or sink wash.

Yes	No

Result: i.e., breathlessness, pain, muscle fatigue, after effects:

Fatigue and Symptom Tracker

Activity: cooking; talking; housework; washing dishes, going out, how many breaks to wash dishes, cook meal, after effects:

____

____

____

____

____

____

____

Notes:____

____

____

____

Use the diagram below to indicate area of pain and/or weakness.

Diagram: B: Muscle burning

N: Numbness

CP: Chest and central back pain

MW: Muscle weakness

S: Stiffness (draw an arrow and write letter for symptom)

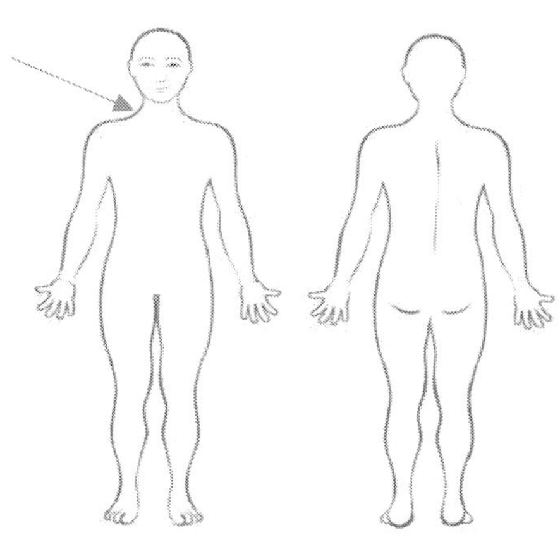

Daily Diary

Day_______________ Date_________

Scale of fatigue 0= fine, 10= extremely tired*: note level of fatigue below during your day*

0---------1---------2----------3---------4--------5----------6---------7--------8--------9---------10

Morning:_______ Afternoon:_______ Evening:_______

<u>Cognitive issues</u>: memory, speech (word forming), comprehension (processing what people are saying)

Write down how it presented itself:

____

____

____

____

____

____

<u>Muscle weakness</u>: jaw, neck, arms (upper/lower), shoulders, lower back/abdomen, hips, legs, swallowing difficulties, head drop:

Activity at time:

____

____

____

____

____

____

<u>Chest and/ or central back pain</u>: activity at time if any; how long it lasted; where exactly and how it presented itself:____

____

____

____

____

____

<u>Shortness of breath</u>: write activity or when lying down; when pulse raised, type of breathlessness:

____
____
____
____
____
____
____

<u>Numbness and tingling/crawling ant sensation</u>: hands; both, one, half, lasted? Feet, toes, lower leg,
other:____
____
____
____
____
____

<u>Balance:</u> try to mark down how often you tipped/wobbled/fell and activity at
time:____
____
____
____
____
____

<u>Bathed: Shower, bath or sink wash.</u>

Yes	No

Result: i.e., breathlessness, pain, muscle fatigue, after effects:____

Daily Diary

Activity: cooking; talking; housework; washing dishes, going out, how many breaks to wash dishes, cook meal, after effects:

____

____

____

____

____

____

____

Notes:____

____

____

____

Use the diagram below to indicate area of pain and/or weakness.

Diagram: B: Muscle burning

N: Numbness

CP: Chest and central back pain

MW: Muscle weakness

S: Stiffness (draw an arrow and write letter for symptom)

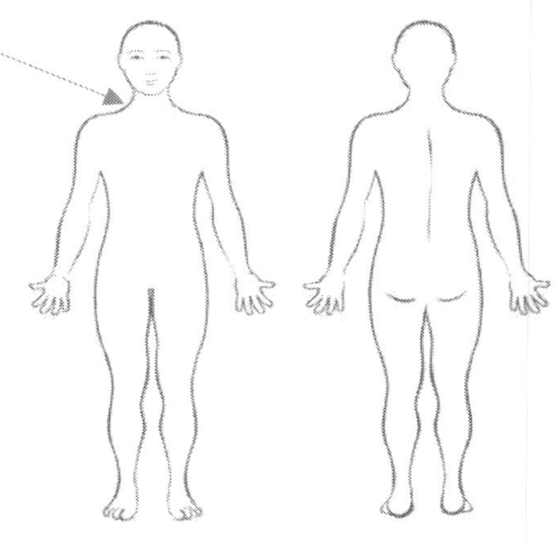

Fatigue and Symptom Tracker

Day________________ Date__________

Scale of fatigue 0= fine, 10= extremely tired*: note level of fatigue below during your day*

0---------1---------2----------3---------4--------5----------6---------7--------8--------9---------10

Morning:_______ Afternoon:_______ Evening:_______

Cognitive issues: memory, speech (word forming), comprehension (processing what people are saying)

Write down how it presented itself:

____

____

____

____

____

____

Muscle weakness: jaw, neck, arms (upper/lower), shoulders, lower back/abdomen, hips, legs, swallowing difficulties, head drop:

Activity at time:

____

____

____

____

____

____

Chest and/ or central back pain: activity at time if any; how long it lasted; where exactly and how it presented itself:____

____

____

____

____

____

Daily Diary

<u>Shortness of breath</u>: write activity or when lying down; when pulse raised, type of breathlessness:

____

Numbness and tingling/crawling ant sensation: hands; both, one, half, lasted? Feet, toes, lower leg, other:

Balance: try to mark down how often you tipped/wobbled/fell and activity at time:

Bathed: Shower, bath or sink wash.

Yes	No

Result: i.e., breathlessness, pain, muscle fatigue, after effects:

<u>Activity</u>: cooking; talking; housework; washing dishes, going out, how many breaks to wash dishes, cook meal, after effects:

____
____
____
____
____
____
____

Notes:____
____
____
____

Use the diagram below to indicate area of pain and/or weakness.

Diagram: B: Muscle burning

N: Numbness

CP: Chest and central back pain

MW: Muscle weakness

S: Stiffness (draw an arrow and write letter for symptom)

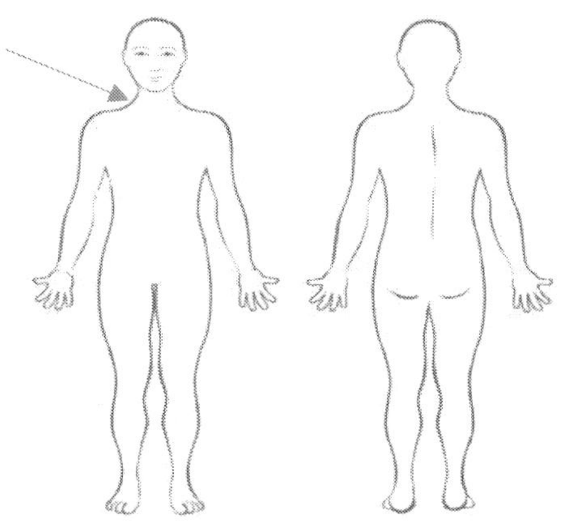

Daily Diary

Day_______________ Date_________

Scale of fatigue 0= fine, 10= extremely tired*: note level of fatigue below during your day*

0---------1---------2----------3---------4--------5----------6---------7--------8--------9---------10

Morning:_______ Afternoon:_______ Evening:_______

Cognitive issues: memory, speech (word forming), comprehension (processing what people are saying)

Write down how it presented itself:

____

____

____

____

____

____

Muscle weakness: jaw, neck, arms (upper/lower), shoulders, lower back/abdomen, hips, legs, swallowing difficulties, head drop:

Activity at time:

____

____

____

____

____

____

Chest and/ or central back pain: activity at time if any; how long it lasted; where exactly and how it presented itself:____

____

____

____

____

____

Shortness of breath: write activity or when lying down; when pulse raised, type of breathlessness:

____

____

____

____

____

____

____

Numbness and tingling/crawling ant sensation: hands; both, one, half, lasted? Feet, toes, lower leg,
other:____

____

____

____

____

____

Balance: try to mark down how often you tipped/wobbled/fell and activity at
time:____

____

____

____

____

____

Bathed: Shower, bath or sink wash.

Yes	No

Result: i.e., breathlessness, pain, muscle fatigue, after
effects:____

Daily Diary

<u>Activity</u>: cooking; talking; housework; washing dishes, going out, how many breaks to wash dishes, cook meal, after effects:

____

____

____

____

____

____

____

Notes:____

____

____

____

Use the diagram below to indicate area of pain and/or weakness.

Diagram: B: Muscle burning

N: Numbness

CP: Chest and central back pain

MW: Muscle weakness

S: Stiffness (draw an arrow and write letter for symptom)

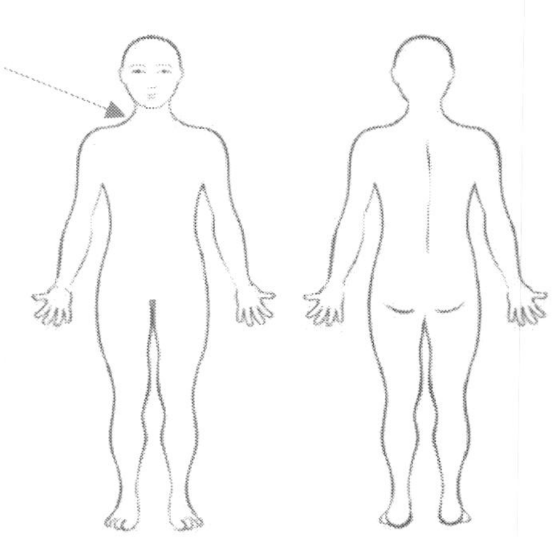

Fatigue and Symptom Tracker

Day________________ Date__________

Scale of fatigue 0= fine, 10= extremely tired*: note level of fatigue below during your day*

0---------1---------2----------3---------4--------5----------6---------7--------8--------9---------10

Morning:________ Afternoon:________ Evening:________

Cognitive issues: memory, speech (word forming), comprehension (processing what people are saying)

Write down how it presented itself:

____

____

____

____

____

____

Muscle weakness: jaw, neck, arms (upper/lower), shoulders, lower back/abdomen, hips, legs, swallowing difficulties, head drop:

Activity at time:

____

____

____

____

____

____

Chest and/ or central back pain: activity at time if any; how long it lasted; where exactly and how it presented itself:____

____

____

____

____

____

Daily Diary

Shortness of breath: write activity or when lying down; when pulse raised, type of breathlessness:

Numbness and tingling/crawling ant sensation: hands; both, one, half, lasted? Feet, toes, lower leg, other:

Balance: try to mark down how often you tipped/wobbled/fell and activity at time:

Bathed: Shower, bath or sink wash.

Yes	No

Result: i.e., breathlessness, pain, muscle fatigue, after effects:

Fatigue and Symptom Tracker

<u>Activity</u>: cooking; talking; housework; washing dishes, going out, how many breaks to wash dishes, cook meal, after effects:

____

____

____

____

____

____

____

Notes:____

____

____

____

Use the diagram below to indicate area of pain and/or weakness.

Diagram: B: Muscle burning

N: Numbness

CP: Chest and central back pain

MW: Muscle weakness

S: Stiffness (draw an arrow and write letter for symptom)

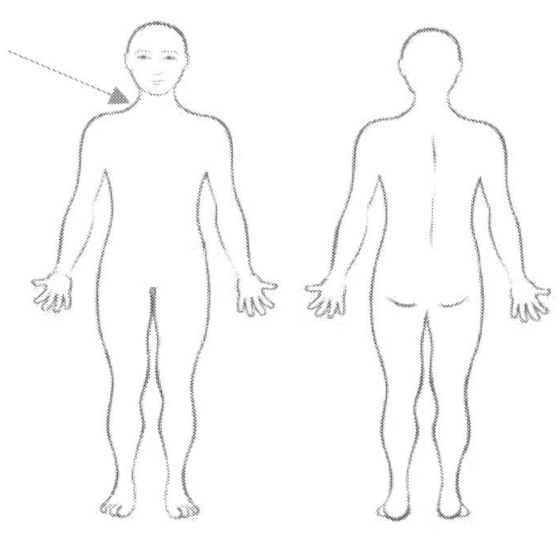

Daily Diary

Day________________ Date__________

Scale of fatigue 0= fine, 10= extremely tired*: note level of fatigue below during your day*

0---------1---------2----------3---------4--------5----------6---------7--------8--------9---------10

Morning:_______ Afternoon:_______ Evening:_______

<u>Cognitive issues</u>: memory, speech (word forming), comprehension (processing what people are saying)

Write down how it presented itself:

____

____

____

____

____

____

<u>Muscle weakness</u>: jaw, neck, arms (upper/lower), shoulders, lower back/abdomen, hips, legs, swallowing difficulties, head drop:

Activity at time:

____

____

____

____

____

____

<u>Chest and/ or central back pain</u>: activity at time if any; how long it lasted; where exactly and how it presented itself:____

____

____

____

____

____

Shortness of breath: write activity or when lying down; when pulse raised, type of breathlessness:

____

____

____

____

____

____

____

Numbness and tingling/crawling ant sensation: hands; both, one, half, lasted? Feet, toes, lower leg, other:__________________________________

____

____

____

____

____

Balance: try to mark down how often you tipped/wobbled/fell and activity at time:__________________________________

____

____

____

____

____

Bathed: Shower, bath or sink wash.

Yes	No

Result: i.e., breathlessness, pain, muscle fatigue, after effects:__________________________________

Daily Diary

Activity: cooking; talking; housework; washing dishes, going out, how many breaks to wash dishes, cook meal, after effects:

____

____

____

____

____

____

____

Notes:____

____

____

____

Use the diagram below to indicate area of pain and/or weakness.

Diagram: B: Muscle burning

N: Numbness

CP: Chest and central back pain

MW: Muscle weakness

S: Stiffness (draw an arrow and write letter for symptom)

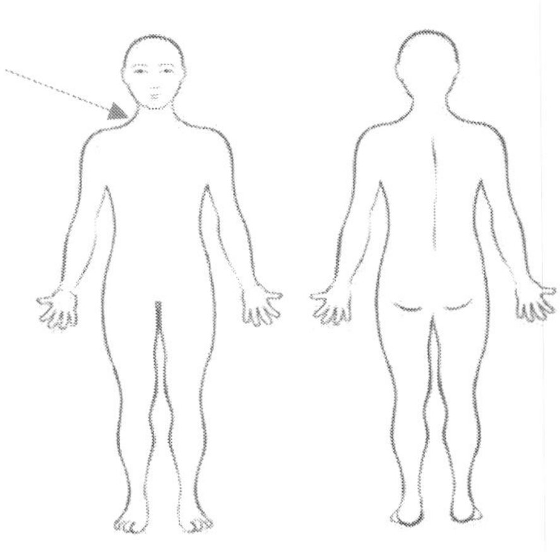

Fatigue and Symptom Tracker

Day________________ Date__________

Scale of fatigue 0= fine, 10= extremely tired*: note level of fatigue below during your day*

0---------1---------2----------3---------4--------5----------6---------7--------8--------9---------10

Morning:_______ Afternoon:_______ Evening:_______

Cognitive issues: memory, speech (word forming), comprehension (processing what people are saying)

Write down how it presented itself:

____

____

____

____

____

____

Muscle weakness: jaw, neck, arms (upper/lower), shoulders, lower back/abdomen, hips, legs, swallowing difficulties, head drop:

Activity at time:

____

____

____

____

____

____

Chest and/ or central back pain: activity at time if any; how long it lasted; where exactly and how it presented itself:____

____

____

____

____

____

Daily Diary

Shortness of breath: write activity or when lying down; when pulse raised, type of breathlessness:

____

Numbness and tingling/crawling ant sensation: hands; both, one, half, lasted? Feet, toes, lower leg, other:________________________________

Balance: try to mark down how often you tipped/wobbled/fell and activity at time:________________________________

Bathed: Shower, bath or sink wash.

Yes	No

Result: i.e., breathlessness, pain, muscle fatigue, after effects:________________________________

Fatigue and Symptom Tracker

Activity: cooking; talking; housework; washing dishes, going out, how many breaks to wash dishes, cook meal, after effects:

____

____

____

____

____

____

____

Notes:____

____

____

____

Use the diagram below to indicate area of pain and/or weakness.

Diagram: B: Muscle burning

N: Numbness

CP: Chest and central back pain

MW: Muscle weakness

S: Stiffness (draw an arrow and write letter for symptom)

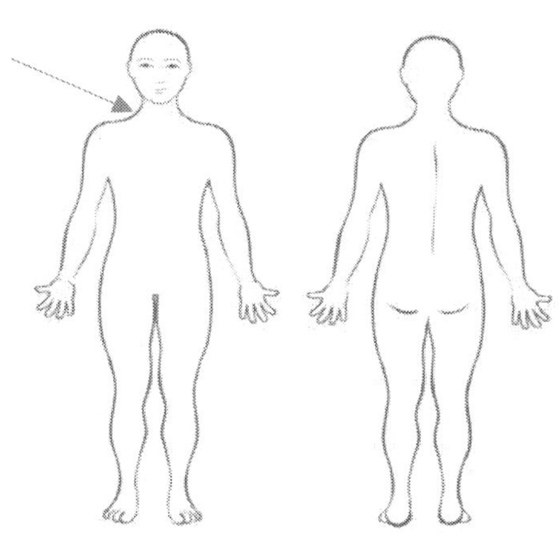

Daily Diary

Day________________ Date__________

Scale of fatigue 0= fine, 10= extremely tired*: note level of fatigue below during your day*

0---------1---------2----------3---------4--------5----------6---------7--------8--------9---------10

Morning:________ Afternoon:________ Evening:________

Cognitive issues: memory, speech (word forming), comprehension (processing what people are saying)

Write down how it presented itself:

Muscle weakness: jaw, neck, arms (upper/lower), shoulders, lower back/abdomen, hips, legs, swallowing difficulties, head drop:

Activity at time:

Chest and/ or central back pain: activity at time if any; how long it lasted; where exactly and how it presented itself:

Shortness of breath: write activity or when lying down; when pulse raised, type of breathlessness:

____

____

____

____

____

____

____

Numbness and tingling/crawling ant sensation: hands; both, one, half, lasted? Feet, toes, lower leg, other:____

____

____

____

____

____

Balance: try to mark down how often you tipped/wobbled/fell and activity at time:____

____

____

____

____

____

Bathed: Shower, bath or sink wash.

Yes	No

Result: i.e., breathlessness, pain, muscle fatigue, after effects:____

Daily Diary

<u>Activity</u>: cooking; talking; housework; washing dishes, going out, how many breaks to wash dishes, cook meal, after effects:

____

____

____

____

____

____

____

Notes:____

____

____

____

Use the diagram below to indicate area of pain and/or weakness.

Diagram: B: Muscle burning

N: Numbness

CP: Chest and central back pain

MW: Muscle weakness

S: Stiffness (draw an arrow and write letter for symptom)

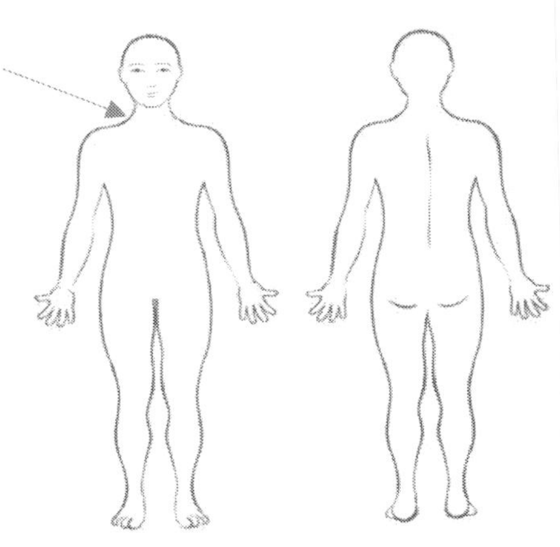

Fatigue and Symptom Tracker

Day________________ Date__________

Scale of fatigue 0= fine, 10= extremely tired*: note level of fatigue below during your day*

0---------1---------2----------3---------4--------5----------6---------7--------8--------9---------10

Morning:________ Afternoon:________ Evening:________

Cognitive issues: memory, speech (word forming), comprehension (processing what people are saying)

Write down how it presented itself:

____

____

____

____

____

____

Muscle weakness: jaw, neck, arms (upper/lower), shoulders, lower back/abdomen, hips, legs, swallowing difficulties, head drop:

Activity at time:

____

____

____

____

____

____

Chest and/ or central back pain: activity at time if any; how long it lasted; where exactly and how it presented itself:____

____

____

____

____

____

Daily Diary

Shortness of breath: write activity or when lying down; when pulse raised, type of breathlessness:

____

Numbness and tingling/crawling ant sensation: hands; both, one, half, lasted? Feet, toes, lower leg, other:

Balance: try to mark down how often you tipped/wobbled/fell and activity at time:

Bathed: Shower, bath or sink wash.

Yes	No

Result: i.e., breathlessness, pain, muscle fatigue, after effects:

Fatigue and Symptom Tracker

Activity: cooking; talking; housework; washing dishes, going out, how many breaks to wash dishes, cook meal, after effects:

____

____

____

____

____

____

____

Notes:____

____

____

____

Use the diagram below to indicate area of pain and/or weakness.

Diagram: B: Muscle burning

N: Numbness

CP: Chest and central back pain

MW: Muscle weakness

S: Stiffness (draw an arrow and write letter for symptom)

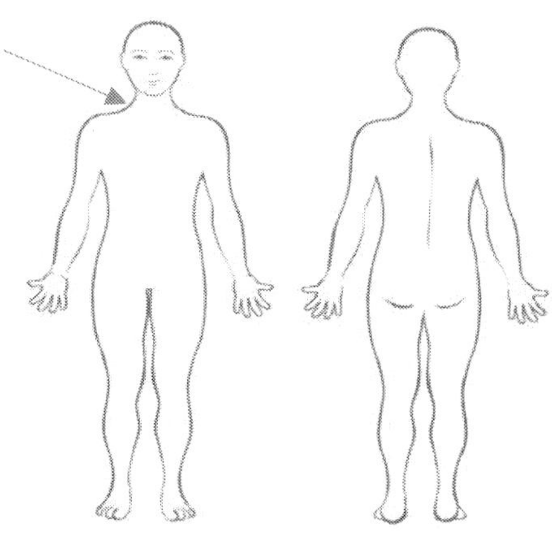

Daily Diary

Day______________ Date________

Scale of fatigue 0= fine, 10= extremely tired*: note level of fatigue below during your day*

0---------1---------2----------3---------4--------5----------6---------7--------8--------9---------10

Morning:_______ Afternoon:_______ Evening:_______

<u>Cognitive issues</u>: memory, speech (word forming), comprehension (processing what people are saying)

Write down how it presented itself:

____

____

____

____

____

____

<u>Muscle weakness</u>: jaw, neck, arms (upper/lower), shoulders, lower back/abdomen, hips, legs, swallowing difficulties, head drop:

Activity at time:

____

____

____

____

____

____

<u>Chest and/ or central back pain</u>: activity at time if any; how long it lasted; where exactly and how it presented itself:____

____

____

____

____

____

Shortness of breath: write activity or when lying down; when pulse raised, type of breathlessness:

____

____

____

____

____

____

____

Numbness and tingling/crawling ant sensation: hands; both, one, half, lasted? Feet, toes, lower leg, other:____

____

____

____

____

____

Balance: try to mark down how often you tipped/wobbled/fell and activity at time:____

____

____

____

____

____

Bathed: Shower, bath or sink wash.

Yes	No

Result: i.e., breathlessness, pain, muscle fatigue, after effects:____

Daily Diary

Activity: cooking; talking; housework; washing dishes, going out, how many breaks to wash dishes, cook meal, after effects:

Notes:

Use the diagram below to indicate area of pain and/or weakness.

Diagram: B: Muscle burning

N: Numbness

CP: Chest and central back pain

MW: Muscle weakness

S: Stiffness (draw an arrow and write letter for symptom)

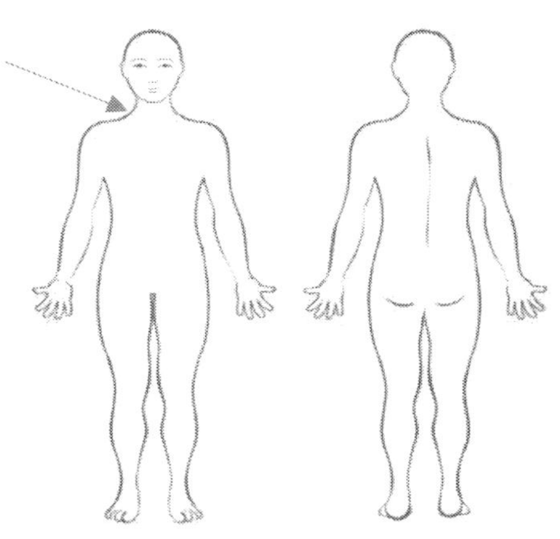

Fatigue and Symptom Tracker

Day________________ Date_________

Scale of fatigue 0= fine, 10= extremely tired*: note level of fatigue below during your day*

0---------1---------2----------3---------4--------5----------6---------7--------8--------9---------10

Morning:_______ Afternoon:_______ Evening:_______

<u>Cognitive issues</u>: memory, speech (word forming), comprehension (processing what people are saying)

Write down how it presented itself:

____

____

____

____

____

____

<u>Muscle weakness</u>: jaw, neck, arms (upper/lower), shoulders, lower back/abdomen, hips, legs, swallowing difficulties, head drop:

Activity at time:

____

____

____

____

____

____

<u>Chest and/ or central back pain</u>: activity at time if any; how long it lasted; where exactly and how it presented itself:____

____

____

____

____

____

Daily Diary

Shortness of breath: write activity or when lying down; when pulse raised, type of breathlessness:

____

____

____

____

____

____

____

Numbness and tingling/crawling ant sensation: hands; both, one, half, lasted? Feet, toes, lower leg, other:____

____

____

____

____

____

Balance: try to mark down how often you tipped/wobbled/fell and activity at time:____

____

____

____

____

____

Bathed: Shower, bath or sink wash.

Yes	No

Result: i.e., breathlessness, pain, muscle fatigue, after effects:____

Fatigue and Symptom Tracker

Activity: cooking; talking; housework; washing dishes, going out, how many breaks to wash dishes, cook meal, after effects:

____

Notes:____________________________________

Use the diagram below to indicate area of pain and/or weakness.

Diagram: B: Muscle burning

N: Numbness

CP: Chest and central back pain

MW: Muscle weakness

S: Stiffness (draw an arrow and write letter for symptom)

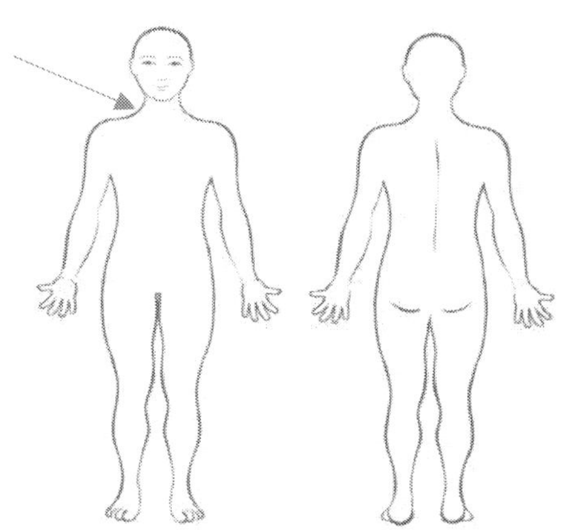

Daily Diary

Day________________ Date__________

Scale of fatigue 0= fine, 10= extremely tired*: note level of fatigue below during your day*

0---------1---------2----------3---------4--------5----------6---------7--------8--------9---------10

Morning:_______ Afternoon:_______ Evening:_______

Cognitive issues: memory, speech (word forming), comprehension (processing what people are saying)

Write down how it presented itself:

Muscle weakness: jaw, neck, arms (upper/lower), shoulders, lower back/abdomen, hips, legs, swallowing difficulties, head drop:

Activity at time:

Chest and/ or central back pain: activity at time if any; how long it lasted; where exactly and how it presented itself:

<u>Shortness of breath</u>: write activity or when lying down; when pulse raised, type of breathlessness:

____

____

____

____

____

____

____

<u>Numbness and tingling/crawling ant sensation</u>: hands; both, one, half, lasted? Feet, toes, lower leg,
other:____

____

____

____

____

____

<u>Balance:</u> try to mark down how often you tipped/wobbled/fell and activity at
time:____

____

____

____

____

____

<u>Bathed: Shower, bath or sink wash.</u>

Yes	No

Result: i.e., breathlessness, pain, muscle fatigue, after
effects:_______________________________________

Daily Diary

<u>Activity</u>: cooking; talking; housework; washing dishes, going out, how many breaks to wash dishes, cook meal, after effects:

____

____

____

____

____

____

____

Notes:____________________________________

____

____

____

Use the diagram below to indicate area of pain and/or weakness.

Diagram: B: Muscle burning

N: Numbness

CP: Chest and central back pain

MW: Muscle weakness

S: Stiffness (draw an arrow and write letter for symptom)

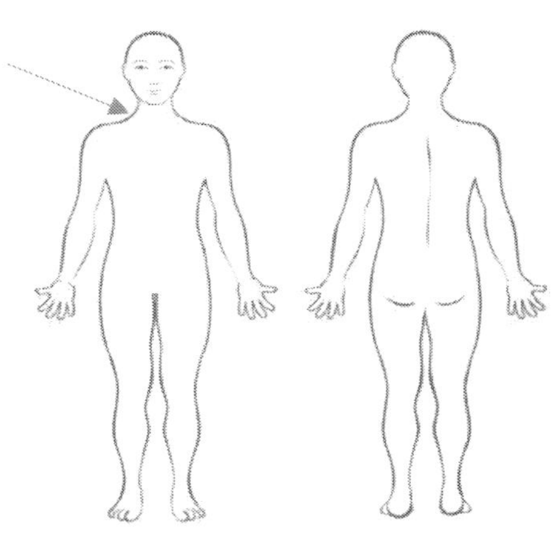

Fatigue and Symptom Tracker

Day_______________ Date_________

Scale of fatigue 0= fine, 10= extremely tired*: note level of fatigue below during your day*

0---------1---------2----------3---------4--------5----------6---------7--------8--------9---------10

Morning:_______ Afternoon:_______ Evening:_______

Cognitive issues: memory, speech (word forming), comprehension (processing what people are saying)

Write down how it presented itself:

____

____

____

____

____

____

Muscle weakness: jaw, neck, arms (upper/lower), shoulders, lower back/abdomen, hips, legs, swallowing difficulties, head drop:

Activity at time:

____

____

____

____

____

____

Chest and/ or central back pain: activity at time if any; how long it lasted; where exactly and how it presented itself:____

____

____

____

____

____

Daily Diary

Shortness of breath: write activity or when lying down; when pulse raised, type of breathlessness:

____

Numbness and tingling/crawling ant sensation: hands; both, one, half, lasted? Feet, toes, lower leg, other:____________________________________

Balance: try to mark down how often you tipped/wobbled/fell and activity at time:____________________________________

Bathed: Shower, bath or sink wash.

Yes	No

Result: i.e., breathlessness, pain, muscle fatigue, after effects:____________________________________

Fatigue and Symptom Tracker

Activity: cooking; talking; housework; washing dishes, going out, how many breaks to wash dishes, cook meal, after effects:

____

____

____

____

____

____

____

Notes:____

____

____

____

Use the diagram below to indicate area of pain and/or weakness.

Diagram: B: Muscle burning

N: Numbness

CP: Chest and central back pain

MW: Muscle weakness

S: Stiffness (draw an arrow and write letter for symptom)

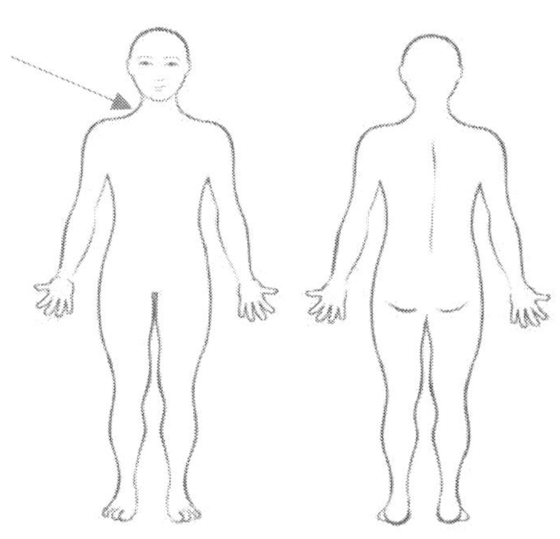

Daily Diary

Day________________ Date__________

Scale of fatigue 0= fine, 10= extremely tired*: note level of fatigue below during your day*

0---------1---------2----------3---------4--------5----------6---------7--------8--------9---------10

Morning:________ Afternoon:________ Evening:________

Cognitive issues: memory, speech (word forming), comprehension (processing what people are saying)

Write down how it presented itself:

____

____

____

____

____

____

Muscle weakness: jaw, neck, arms (upper/lower), shoulders, lower back/abdomen, hips, legs, swallowing difficulties, head drop:

Activity at time:

____

____

____

____

____

____

Chest and/ or central back pain: activity at time if any; how long it lasted; where exactly and how it presented itself:____

____

____

____

____

____

Shortness of breath: write activity or when lying down; when pulse raised, type of breathlessness:

____

Numbness and tingling/crawling ant sensation: hands; both, one, half, lasted? Feet, toes, lower leg, other:____

Balance: try to mark down how often you tipped/wobbled/fell and activity at time:____

Bathed: Shower, bath or sink wash.

Yes	No

Result: i.e., breathlessness, pain, muscle fatigue, after effects:____

Daily Diary

Activity: cooking; talking; housework; washing dishes, going out, how many breaks to wash dishes, cook meal, after effects:

____

____

____

____

____

____

____

Notes:____

____

____

____

Use the diagram below to indicate area of pain and/or weakness.

Diagram: B: Muscle burning

N: Numbness

CP: Chest and central back pain

MW: Muscle weakness

S: Stiffness (draw an arrow and write letter for symptom)

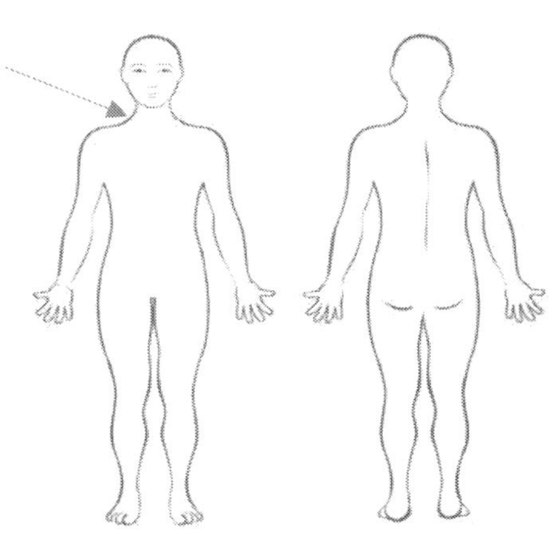

Fatigue and Symptom Tracker

Day________________ Date_________

Scale of fatigue 0= fine, 10= extremely tired*: note level of fatigue below during your day*

0---------1---------2----------3---------4--------5----------6---------7--------8--------9---------10

Morning:_______ Afternoon:_______ Evening:_______

Cognitive issues: memory, speech (word forming), comprehension (processing what people are saying)

Write down how it presented itself:

____

____

____

____

____

____

Muscle weakness: jaw, neck, arms (upper/lower), shoulders, lower back/abdomen, hips, legs, swallowing difficulties, head drop:

Activity at time:

____

____

____

____

____

____

Chest and/ or central back pain: activity at time if any; how long it lasted; where exactly and how it presented itself:____

____

____

____

____

____

Daily Diary

Shortness of breath: write activity or when lying down; when pulse raised, type of breathlessness:

____
____
____
____
____
____
____

Numbness and tingling/crawling ant sensation: hands; both, one, half, lasted? Feet, toes, lower leg, other:______________________________________

____
____
____
____
____

Balance: try to mark down how often you tipped/wobbled/fell and activity at time:______________________________________

____
____
____
____
____

Bathed: Shower, bath or sink wash.

Yes	No

Result: i.e., breathlessness, pain, muscle fatigue, after effects:______________________________________

Fatigue and Symptom Tracker

<u>Activity</u>: cooking; talking; housework; washing dishes, going out, how many breaks to wash dishes, cook meal, after effects:

____

____

____

____

____

____

____

Notes:____

____

____

____

Use the diagram below to indicate area of pain and/or weakness.

Diagram: B: Muscle burning

N: Numbness

CP: Chest and central back pain

MW: Muscle weakness

S: Stiffness (draw an arrow and write letter for symptom)

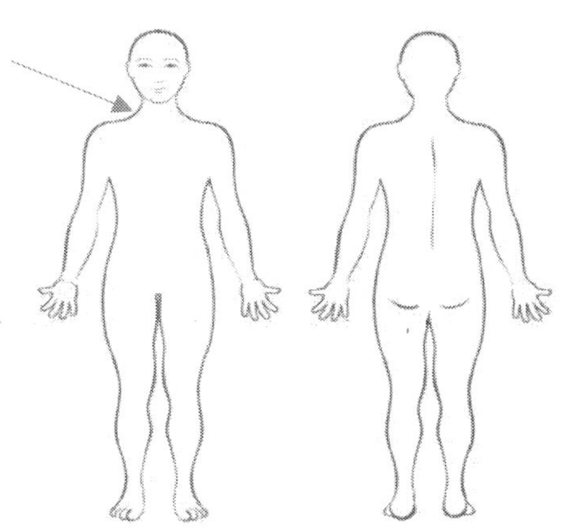

I hope the use of this Journal has enabled you to have a clearer idea of which activities aggravate and alleviate your condition. It should also become a handy diary to take along to your medical practitioner to enable you to have a fuller picture of your symptoms so that you don't forget to mention them if needed. Tracking your health, activity and medication can assist in building a picture of how to manage your day to day activities and therapies.

We have all probably experienced the frustration of leaving a possibly, long awaited appointment realising we had forgotten to tell the Doctor important information. These lapses in memory can be due to pain, fatigue or cognitive issues so having it written down with body diagrams can be very helpful. The note section can include which, if any, medications alleviate your symptoms.

Chronic fluctuating health conditions like Lupus, CFS, MS, Fibromyalgia and ME can present with many symptoms, especially in the moderate to severe cases as well as the milder cases. Taking notes as and when they occur can help present a full picture of how your illness is progressing (for better or worse) and how it impacts your daily life and functioning.

For those in need of disability benefits or insurance assistance, this diary may be of assistance to refer to as a comprehensive record of your daily experiences.

I have found it very useful to refer to during my medical appointments and in relation to applying for assistance relating to disability.

I wish you all good health for the future.

Printed in Great Britain
by Amazon